Dash Diet Recipe Collection

The Most Comprehensive mix of Dash Diet
Recipes to enjoy your everyday meals

Natalie Puckett

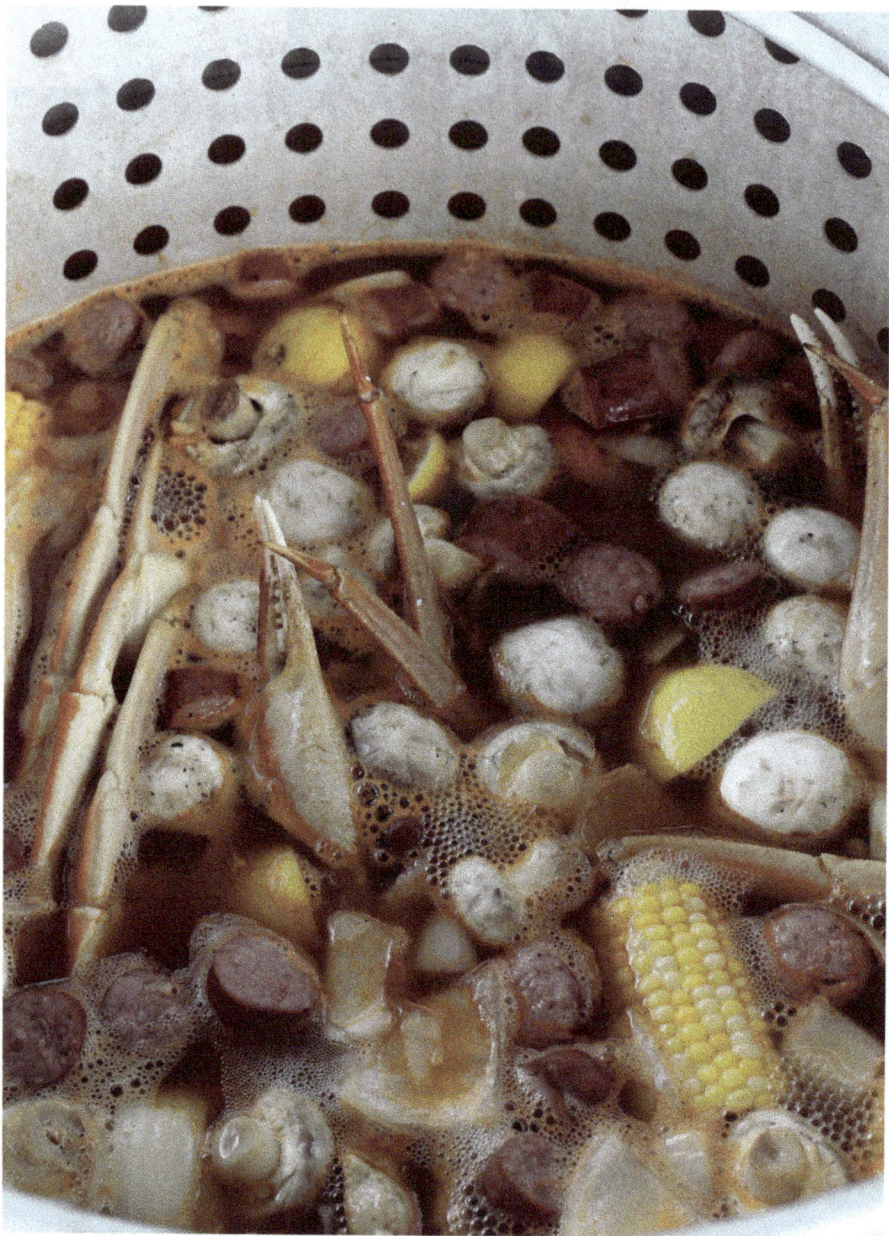

Table of Contents

Cajun Snow Crab

Serving: 2

 Prep Time: 10 minutes

Cook Time: 10 minutes

Ingredients:

1 lemon, fresh and quartered tablespoons

Cajun seasoning

Bay leaves

Snow crab legs, precooked and defrosted Golden ghee

How To:

1.   Take a large pot and fill it about halfway with sunflower seeds and water.

2.   Bring the water to a boil.

3.   Squeeze lemon juice into the pot and toss in remaining lemon quarters.

4.   Add bay leaves and Cajun seasoning.

5.   Season for 1 minute.

6.   Add crab legs and boil for 8 minutes (make sure to keep them submerged the whole time).

7.   Melt ghee in microwave and use as dipping sauce, enjoy!

Nutrition (Per Serving)

Calories: 643

Fat: 51g

Carbohydrates: 3g

Protein: 41g

Grilled Lime Shrimp

Serving: 8

Prep Time: 25 minutes

Cook Time: 5 minutes

Ingredients:

1-pound medium shrimp, peeled and deveined

1 lime, juiced

½ cup olive oil

Cajun seasoning

How To:

1.   Take a re-sealable zip bag and add lime juice, Cajun seasoning, olive oil.

2.   Add shrimp and shake it well, let it marinate for 20 minutes.

3.   Pre-heat your outdoor grill to medium heat.

4.   Lightly grease the grate.

5.   Remove shrimp from marinade and cook for 2 minutes per side.

6.   Serve and enjoy!

Nutrition (Per Serving)

Calories: 188

Fat: 3g

Net Carbohydrates: 1.2g

Protein: 13g

Calamari Citrus

Serving: 4

Prep Time: 10 minutes

Cook Time: 5 minutes

Ingredients:

1 lime, sliced

lemon, sliced

Pounds calamari tubes and tentacles, sliced

Pepper to taste

¼ cup olive oil

garlic cloves, minced

tablespoons lemon juice

orange, peeled and cut into segments

tablespoons cilantro, chopped

How To:

1.   Take a bowl and add calamari, pepper, lime slices, lemon slices, orange slices, garlic, oil, cilantro, lemon juice and toss well.

2.   Take a pan and place it over medium-high heat.

3.   Add calamari mix and cook for 5 minutes.

4.   Divide into bowls and serve.

5.   Enjoy!

Nutrition (Per Serving)

Calories: 190

Fat: 2g

Net Carbohydrates: 11g

Protein: 14g

Baked Chicken

Prep time: 10 minutes

Cook time: 1 hour

Servings: 4

Ingredients

Chicken – 3 to 4 pounds, cut into parts Olive oil – 3 Tbsp.

Thyme – ½ tsp.

Sea salt – ¼ tsp.

Ground black pepper

Low-sodium chicken stock – ½ cup

Method

1.   Preheat the oven to 400F.

2.   Rub oil over chicken pieces. Sprinkle with salt, thyme, and pepper.

3.   Place chicken in the roasting pan.

4.   Bake in the oven for 30 minutes.

5.   Then lower the heat to 350F.

6.   Bake for 15 to 30 minutes more or until juice runs clear.

7.   Serve.

Nutritional Facts Per Serving

Calories: 550

Fat: 19g

Carb: 0g

Protein: 91g

Sodium 480mg

Orange Chicken and Broccoli Stir-Fry

Prep time: 10 minutes

Cook time: 15 minutes

Servings: 4

Ingredients

Olive oil – 1 Tbsp.

Chicken breast – 1 pound, boneless and skinless, cut into strips
Orange juice – 1/3 cup Homemade soy sauce - 2 Tbsp.

Cornstarch – 2 tsp.

Broccoli – 2 cups, cut into small pieces Snow peas – 1 cup

Cabbage – 2 cups, shredded Brown rice – 2 cups, cooked
Sesame seeds – 1 Tbsp.

Method

1.   Combine the orange juice, soy sauce, and corn starch in a bowl. Set aside.

2.   Heat oil in a pan. Add chicken.

3.   Stir-fry until the chicken is golden brown on all sides, about 5 minutes.

4.   Add snow peas, cabbage, broccoli, and sauce mixture.

5.   Continue to stir-fry for 8 minutes or until vegetables are tender but still crisp.

Nutritional Facts Per Serving

Calories: 340

Fat: 8g

Carb: 35g

Protein: 28g

Sodium 240mg

Mediterranean Lemon Chicken and Potatoes

Prep time: 10 minutes

Cook time: 30 minutes

Servings: 4

Ingredients

Chicken breast – 1 ½ pound, skinless and boneless, cut into 1-inch cubes

Yukon Gold potatoes – 1 pound, cut into cubes

Onion – 1, chopped

Red pepper – 1, chopped

Low-sodium vinaigrette – ½ cup

Lemon juice – ¼ cup Oregano – 1 tsp.

Garlic powder – ½ tsp.

Chopped tomato – ½ cup

Ground black pepper to taste

Method

1.   Preheat oven to 400F.

2.   Except for the tomatoes, mix everything in a bowl.

3.   On 4 aluminum foils, place an equal amount of chicken and potato mixture. Fold to make packets.

4.   Bake at 400F for 30 minutes. Open packets.

5.   Top with chopped tomatoes.

6.   Season with black pepper to taste.

Nutritional Facts Per Serving

Calories: 320

Fat: 4g

Carb: 34g

Protein: 43g

Sodium 420mg

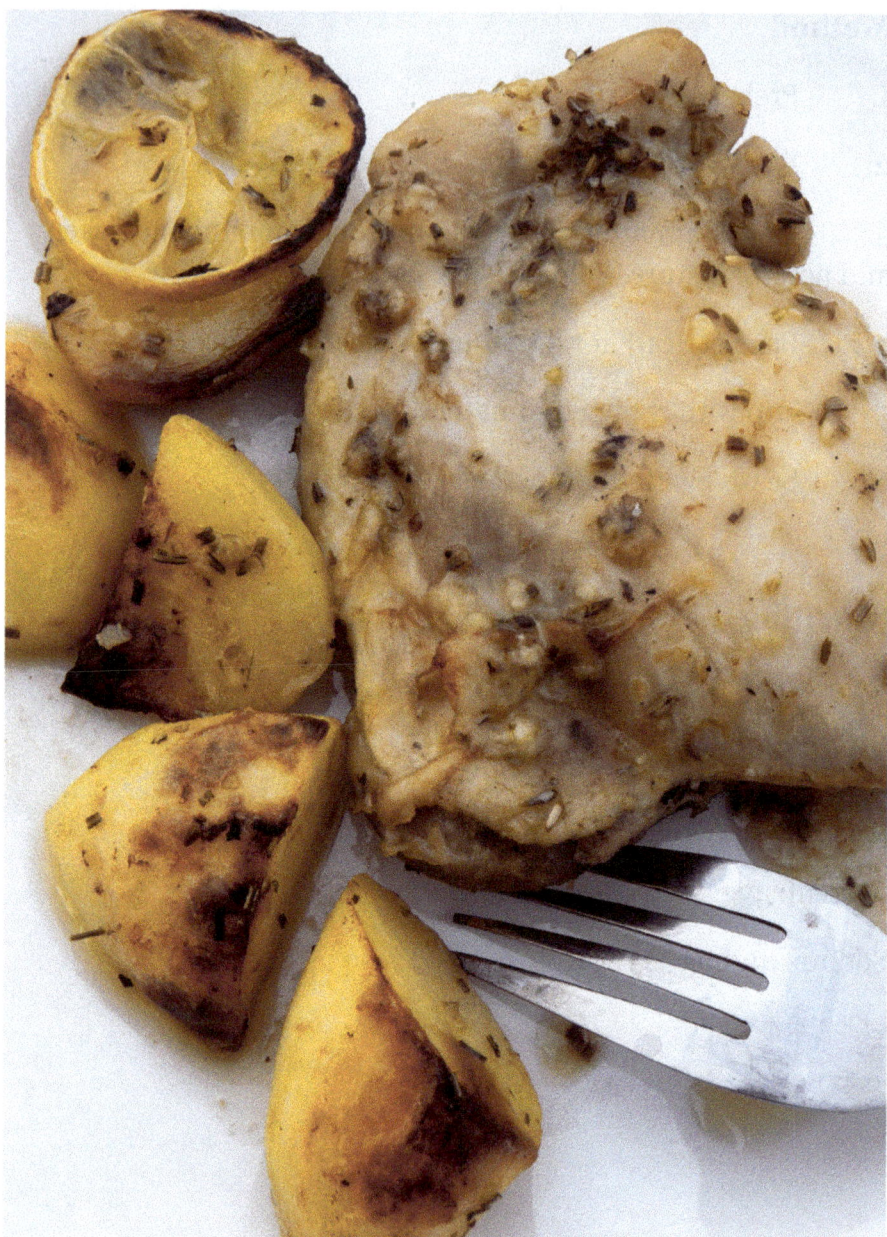

Tandoori Chicken

Prep time: 10 minutes

Cook time: 20 minutes

Servings: 6

Ingredients

Nonfat yogurt – 1 cup, plain

Lemon juice – ½ cup Garlic – 5 cloves, crushed Paprika – 2 Tbsp.

Curry powder – 1 tsp.

Ground ginger – 1 tsp.

Red pepper flakes – 1 tsp.

Chicken breasts – 6, skinless and boneless, cut into 2-inch chunks Wooden skewers – 6, soaked in water

Method

1.   Preheat the oven to 400F.

2.   In a bowl, combine lemon juice, yogurt, garlic, and spices. Blend well.

3.	Divide chicken and thread onto skewers. Place skewers in a baking dish.

4.	Pour half of the yogurt mixture onto chicken. Cover and marinate in the refrigerator for 20 minutes

5.	Spray a baking dish with cooking spray.

6.	Place chicken skewers in the pan and coat with the remaining ½ of yogurt marinade.

7.	Bake in the oven until chicken is cooked, about 15 to 20 minutes.

8.	Serve with veggies or brown rice.

Nutritional Facts Per Serving

Calories: 175

Fat: 2g

Carb: 8g

Protein: 30g

Sodium 105mg

Grilled Chicken Salad

Prep time: 5 minutes

Cook time: 10 minutes

Servings: 4

Ingredients

For the dressing

Red wine vinegar – ½ cup

Garlic – 4 cloves, minced

Extra-virgin olive oil – 1 Tbsp.

Finely chopped red onion – 1 Tbsp.

Finely chopped celery -1 Tbsp. Ground black pepper to taste For the salad

Chicken breasts – 4 (4-ounce each), boneless, skinless

Garlic – 2 cloves

Lettuce leaves - 8 cups

Ripe black olives – 16

Navel oranges – 2, peeled and sliced

Method

1.   To make the dressing, in a bowl, combine all the dressing ingredients mix and keep in the refrigerator.

2.   Heat a gas grill or broiler.

3.   Lightly coat the broiler pan or grill rack with cooking spray.

4.   Position the cooking rack 4 to 6 inches from the heat source.

5.   Rub the chicken breasts with garlic and discard the cloves.

6.   Broil or grill the chicken about 5 minutes per side, or until just cooked through.

7.   Slice the chicken. Arrange with lettuce, olives, and oranges.

8.   Drizzle with dressing and serve.

Nutritional Facts Per Serving

Calories: 237
Fat: 9g
Carb: 12g
Protein: 27g
Sodium 199mg

Hearty Cashew and Almond Butter

Serving: 1 and ½ cups

Prep Time: 5 minutes

Cook Time: Nil

Ingredients:

1 cup almonds, blanched

1/3 cup cashew nuts

2 tablespoons coconut oil

½ teaspoon cinnamon

How To:

1. Pre-heat your oven to 350 degrees F.

2. Bake almonds and cashews for 12 minutes.

3. Let them cool.

4. Transfer to food processor and add remaining ingredients.

5. Add oil and keep blending until smooth.

6. Serve and enjoy!

Nutrition (Per Serving)

Calories: 205

Fat: 19g

Carbohydrates: g

Protein: 2.8g

Red Coleslaw

Serving: 4

Prep Time: 10 minutes

Cook Time: 0 minutes

Ingredients:

1 2/3 pounds red cabbage

2 tablespoons ground caraway seeds

1 tablespoon whole grain mustard

1 1/4 cups mayonnaise, low fat, low sodium Salt and black pepper

How To:

1.   Cut the red cabbage into small slices.

2.   Take a large-sized bowl and add all the ingredients alongside cabbage.

3.   Mix well, season with salt and pepper.

4. Serve and enjoy!

Nutrition (Per Serving)

Calories: 406

Fat: 40.8g

Carbohydrates: 10g

Protein: 2.2g

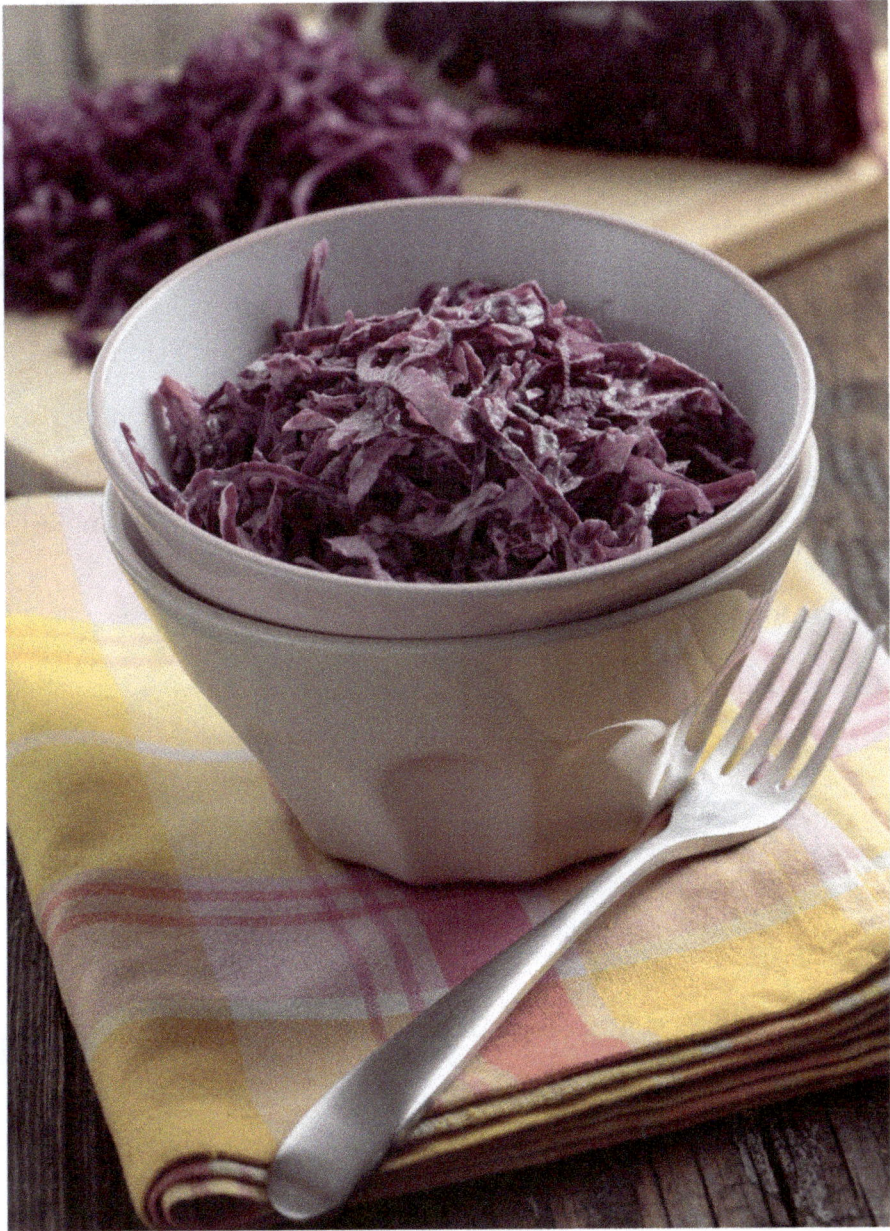

Avocado Mayo Medley

Serving: 4

Prep Time: 5 minutes

Cook Time: Nil

Ingredients:

1 medium avocado, cut into chunks

½ teaspoon ground cayenne pepper

2 tablespoons fresh cilantro

¼ cup olive oil

½ cup mayo, low fat and los sodium

How To:

1.   Take a food processor and add avocado, cayenne pepper, lime juice, salt and cilantro.

2.   Mix until smooth.

3.   Slowly incorporate olive oil, add 1 tablespoon at a time and keep processing between additions.

4.   Store and use as needed!

Nutrition (Per Serving)

Calories: 231

Fat: 20g

Carbohydrates: 5g

Protein: 3g

Amazing Garlic Aioli

Serving: 4

Prep Time: 5 minutes

Cook Time: Nil

Ingredients:

½ cup mayonnaise, low fat and low sodium 2 garlic cloves, minced Juice of 1 lemon

1 tablespoon fresh-flat leaf Italian parsley, chopped

1 teaspoon chives, chopped Salt and pepper to taste

How To:

1.	Add mayonnaise, garlic, parsley, lemon juice, chives and season with salt and pepper.

2.	Blend until combined well.

3.	Pour into refrigerator and chill for 30 minutes.

4.	Serve and use as needed!

Nutrition (Per Serving)

Calories: 813

Fat: 88g

Carbohydrates: 9g

Protein: 2g

Easy Seed Crackers

Serving: 72 crackers

Prep Time: 10 minutes

Cooking Time: 60 minutes

Ingredients:

1 cup boiling water

1/3 cup chia seeds

1/3 cup sesame seeds

1/3 cup pumpkin seeds

1/3 cup Flaxseeds

1/3 cup sunflower seeds

1 tablespoon Psyllium powder

1 cup almond flour

1 teaspoon salt

¼ cup coconut oil, melted

How To:

1.   Pre-heat your oven to 300 degrees F.

2.   Line a cookie sheet with parchment paper and keep it on the side.

3.   Add listed ingredients (except coconut oil and water) to food processor and pulse until ground.

4.   Transfer to a large mixing bowl and pour melted coconut oil and boiling water, mix.

5.   Transfer mix to prepared sheet and spread into a thin layer.

6.   Cut dough into crackers and bake for 60 minutes.

7.   Cool and serve.

8.   Enjoy!

Nutrition (Per Serving)

Total Carbs: 10.6g

Fiber: 3g

Protein: 5g

Fat: 14.6g

Hearty Almond Crackers

Serving: 40 crackers

Prep Time: 10 minutes

Cooking Time: 20 minutes

Ingredients:

1 cup almond flour

¼ teaspoon baking soda

1/8 teaspoon black pepper

3 tablespoons sesame seeds

1 egg, beaten

Salt and pepper to taste

How To:

1.   Pre-heat your oven to 350 degrees F.

2.   Line two baking sheets with parchment paper and keep them on the side.

3.   Mix the dry ingredients in a large bowl and add egg, mix well and form dough.

4. Divide dough into two balls.

5. Roll out the dough between two pieces of parchment paper.

6. Cut into crackers and transfer them to prepared baking sheet.

7. Bake for 15-20 minutes.

8. Repeat until all the dough has been used up.

9. Leave crackers to cool and serve.

10. Enjoy!

Nutrition (Per Serving)

Total Carbs: 8g

Fiber: 2g

Protein: 9g

Fat: 28g

Black Bean Salsa

Serving: 4

Prep Time: 10 minutes

Cook Time: Nil

Ingredients:

1 tablespoon coconut amines

½ teaspoon cumin, ground

1 cup canned black beans, no salt

1 cup salsa

6 cups romaine lettuce, torn

½ cup avocado, peeled, pitted and cubed

How To:

1.   Take a bowl and add beans, alongside other ingredients.

2.   Toss well and serve.

3.   Enjoy!

Nutrition (Per Serving)

Calories: 181

Fat: 5g

Carbohydrates: 14g

Protein: 7g

Delish Pineapple and Coconut Milk Smoothie

Serving: 2

Prep Time: 5 minutes

Ingredients:

¼ cup pineapple, frozen

¾ cup coconut milk

How To:

1.   Add the listed ingredients to blender and blend well on high.

2.   Once the mixture is smooth, pour smoothie in tall glass and serve.

3.   Chill and enjoy!

Nutrition (Per Serving)

Calories: 200

Fat: 10g

Carbohydrates: 14g

Protein 2g

The Minty Refresher

Serving: 2

Prep Time: 5 minutes

Ingredients:

2 cups mint tea

1 cucumber, peeled

2 green apples

1 cup blueberries

Stevia (to sweeten)

Few slices of lime/lemon for garnish

How To:

1.   Add the listed ingredients to your blender and blend until smooth.

2.   Add ice and sweeten with a bit of stevia.

3.   Garnish with lime/lemon slices.

4.   Serve and enjoy!

Nutrition (Per Serving)

Calories: 200

Fat: 10g

Carbohydrates: 14g

Protein 2g

Strawberry and Clementine Glass

Serving: 2

Prep Time: 5 minutes

Ingredients:

8 ounces strawberries, fresh

1 banana, chopped into chunks

2 Clementines/Mandarins

How To:

1.   Peel the clementines and remove seeds.

2.   Add the listed ingredients to your blender/food processor and blend until smooth.

3.   Serve chilled and enjoy!

Nutrition (Per Serving)

Calories: 200

Fat: 10g

Carbohydrates: 14g

Protein 2g

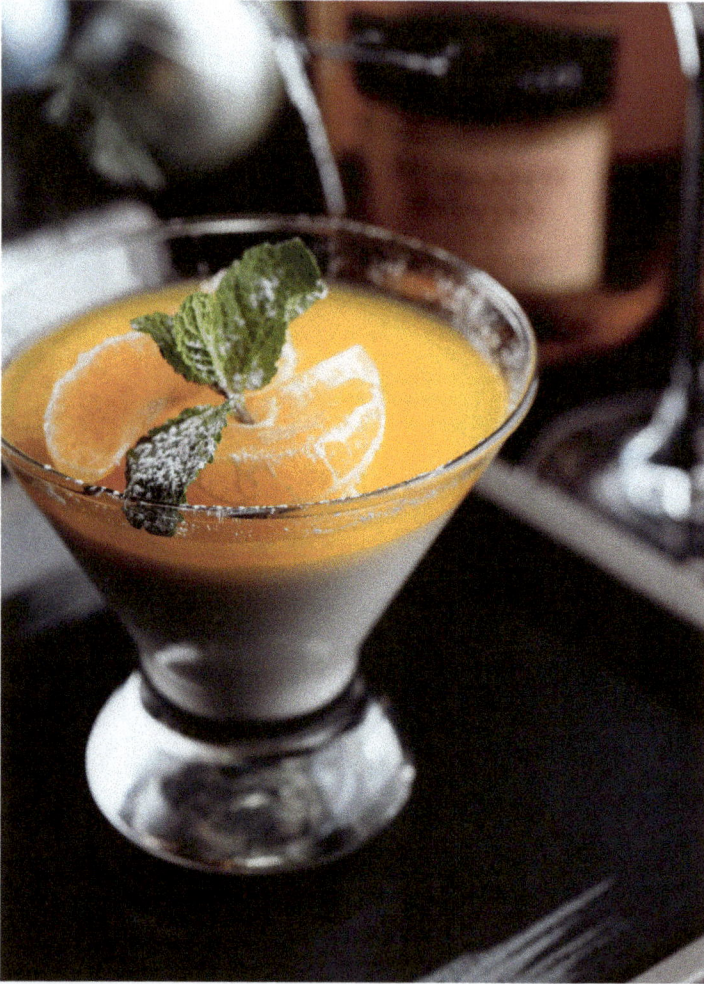

Cabbage and Coconut Chia

Smoothie

Serving: 2

Prep Time: 5 minutes

Ingredients:

1/3 cup cabbage

1 cup cold unsweetened coconut milk

1 tablespoon chia seeds

½ cup cherries

½ cup spinach

How To:

1.   Add coconut milk to your blender.

2.   Cut cabbage and add to your blender.

3.   Place chia seeds in a coffee grinder and chop to powder, brush the powder into the blender.

4.   Pit the cherries and add them to the blender.

5. Wash and dry the spinach and chop.

6. Add to the mix.

7. Cover and blend on low followed by medium.

8. Taste the texture and serve chilled!

Nutrition (Per Serving)

Calories: 200

Fat: 10g

Carbohydrates: 14g

Protein 2g

The Cherry Beet Delight

Serving: 2

Prep Time: 5 minutes

Ingredients:

1 cup cherries, pitted

½ cup beets

Few banana slices

1 cup water, filtered, alkaline

1 cup coconut milk

Pinch of organic vanilla powder

Pinch of cinnamon

Pinch of stevia

Few mint leaves/lime slices to garnish

How To:

1.   Add berries, beets, water, banana slices, coconut milk to your blender.

2.   Blend well until smooth.

3. Add more water if the texture is too creamy for you.

4. Add coconut oil, vanilla, cinnamon and stir.

5. Add a bit of stevia for extra sweetness.

6. Garnish with mint leaves and lime slices.

7. Enjoy!

Nutrition (Per Serving)

Calories: 200

Fat: 10g

Carbohydrates: 14g

Protein 2g

Satisfying Honey and Coconut Porridge

Serving: 8

Prep Time: 10 minutes

Cook Time: 8 hours

Ingredients:

4 cups light coconut milk

3 cups apple juice

2 ¼ cups coconut flour

1 teaspoon ground cinnamon

¼ cup honey

How To:

1.   In a Slow Cooker, add the coconut milk, apple juice, flour, cinnamon and honey.

2.   Stir well.

3.   Close lid and cook on LOW for 8 hours.

4.   Open lid and stir.

5.   Serve with an additional seasoning of fresh fruits.

6.   Enjoy!

Nutrition (Per Serving)

Calories: 372

Fat: 14g

Carbohydrates: 56g

Protein: 8g

Pure Maple Glazed Carrots

Serving: 6

Prep Time: 10 minutes

Cook Time: 8 hours

Ingredients:

¼ cup pure maple syrup

½ teaspoon ground ginger

¼ teaspoon ground nutmeg

½ teaspoon salt

Juice of 1 orange

1-pound baby carrots

How To:

1.   Take a small bowl and whisk in syrup, nutmeg, ginger, salt, orange juice.

2.   Add carrots to your Slow Cooker and pour the maple syrup.

3.   Toss to coat.

4.   Close lid and cook on LOW for 8 hours.

5.   Serve and enjoy!

Nutrition (Per Serving)

Calories: 76

Fat: 1g

Carbohydrates: 19g

Protein: 76g

Ginger and Orange

Serving: 6

Prep Time: 20 minutes

Cook Time: 8 hours

Ingredients:

2 pounds beets, peeled and cut into wedges

Juice of 2 oranges

Zest of 1 orange

1 teaspoon fresh ginger, grated

1 tablespoon honey

1 tablespoon apple cider vinegar

1/8 teaspoon fresh ground black pepper Sea salt

How To:

1.   Add beets, zest, orange juice, ginger, honey, pepper, salt and vinegar to your Slow Cooker.

2.   Stir well.

3.   Close lid and cook on LOW for 8 hours.

4.   Serve and enjoy!

Nutrition (Per Serving)

Calories: 108

Fat: 1g

Carbohydrates: 25g

Protein: 3g

Pineapple Rice

Serving: 2

Prep Time: 10 minutes

Cook Time: 2 hours

Ingredients:

1 cup rice

2 cups water

1 small cauliflower, florets separated and chopped ½ small pineapple, peeled and chopped Salt and pepper as needed

1 teaspoon olive oil

How To:

1.   Add rice, cauliflower, pineapple, water, oil, salt and pepper to your Slow Cooker.

2.   Gently stir.

3.   Place lid and cook on HIGH for 2 hours.

4.   Fluff the rice with fork and season with more salt and pepper if needed.

5.   Divide between serving platters and enjoy!

Nutrition (Per Serving)

Calories: 152

Fat: 4g

Carbohydrates: 18g

Protein: 4g

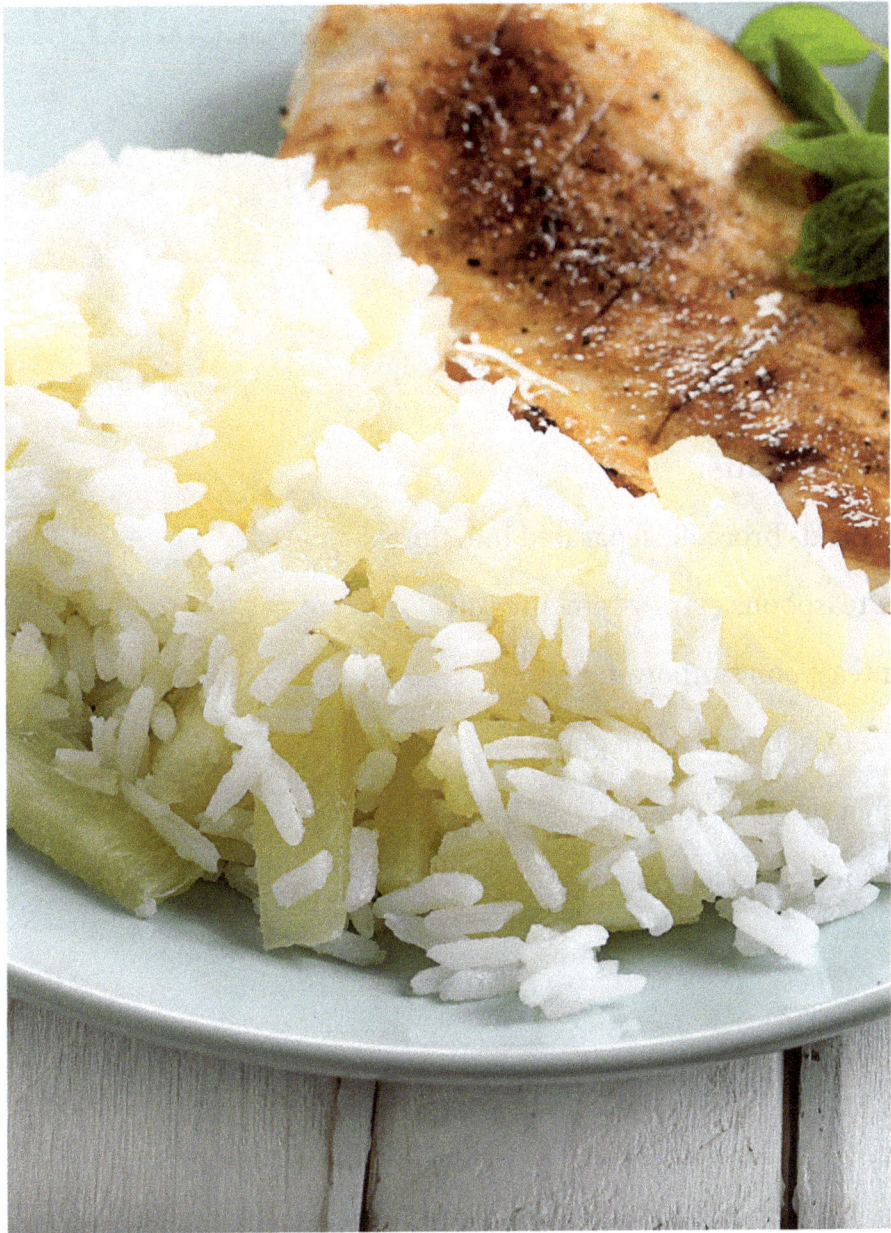

Creative Lemon and Broccoli Dish

Serving: 6

Prep Time: 10 minutes

Cook Time: 15 minutes

Ingredients:

2 heads broccoli, separated into florets

2 teaspoons extra virgin olive oil

1 teaspoon sunflower seeds

½ teaspoon black pepper

1 garlic clove, minced

½ teaspoon lemon juice

How To:

1.   Pre-heat your oven to 400 degrees F.

2.   Take a large sized bowl and add broccoli florets.

3.   Drizzle olive oil and season with pepper, sunflower seeds and garlic.

4.   Spread broccoli out in a single even layer on a baking sheet.

5.   Bake for 15-20 minutes until fork tender.

6.   Squeeze lemon juice on top.

7. Serve and enjoy!

Nutrition (Per Serving)

Calories: 49

Fat: 1.9g

Carbohydrates: 7g

Protein: 3g

Herbed Parmesan Walnuts

Serving: 4

Prep Time: 5 minutes

Cook Time: 30 minutes

Ingredients:

½ cup kite ricotta/cashew cheese

½ teaspoon Italian herb seasoning and garlic sunflower seeds

1 teaspoon parsley flakes

2 cups walnuts

1 egg white

How To:

1.   Preheat your oven to 250 degrees F.

2.   Take a bowl and add all ingredients except the albumen and walnuts.

3.   Whisk within the albumen, stir in halved walnuts and blend well.

4.   Transfer the mixture to a greased baking sheet and bake for half-hour.

5.   Serve and enjoy!

Nutrition (Per Serving)

Calories: 220

Fat: 21g

Carbohydrates: 4g

Protein 8g

Amazing Scrambled Turkey Eggs

Serving: 2

Prep Time: 15 minutes

Cook Time: 15 minutes

Ingredients:

1 tablespoon coconut oil

1 medium red bell pepper, diced

½ medium yellow onion, diced

¼ teaspoon hot pepper sauce

3 large free-range eggs

¼ teaspoon black pepper, freshly ground ¼ teaspoon salt

How To:

1.   Set a pan to medium-high heat, add copra oil, let it heat up.

2.   Add onions and sauté.

3.   Add turkey and red pepper.

4.   Cook until the turkey is cooked.

5.   Take a bowl and beat eggs, stir in salt and pepper.

6.   Pour eggs within the pan with turkey and gently cook and scramble eggs.

7.   Top with sauce and enjoy!

Nutrition (Per Serving)

Calories: 435

Fat: 30g

Carbohydrates: 34g

Protein: 16g

Egg and Bacon Cups

Serving: 6

Prep Time: 10 minutes

Cook Time: 15 minutes

Ingredients:

2 bacon strips

2 large eggs

A handful of fresh spinach

¼ cup cheese

Salt and pepper to taste

How To:

1.   Preheat your oven to 400 degrees F.

2.   Fry bacon during a skillet over medium heat, drain the oil and keep them on the side.

3.   Take muffin tin and grease with oil.

4.   Line with a slice of bacon, depress the bacon well, ensuring that the ends are protruding (to be used as handles).

5.   Take a bowl and beat eggs.

6.   Drain and pat the spinach dry.

7.   Add the spinach to the eggs.

8.   Add 1 / 4 of the mixture in each of your muffin tins.

9.   Sprinkle cheese and season.

10.   Bake for quarter-hour.

11.   Enjoy!

Nutrition (Per Serving)

Calories: 101

Fat: 7g

Carbohydrates: 2g

Protein: 8g

Fiber: 1g

Net Carbs: 1g

Pepperoni Omelet

Serving: 2

Prep Time: 5 minutes

Cook Time: 20 minutes

Ingredients:

3 eggs

7 pepperoni slices

1 teaspoon coconut cream

Salt and freshly ground black pepper, to taste 1 tablespoons butter

How To:

1.   Take a bowl and whisk eggs with all the remaining ingredients in it.

2.   Then take a skillet and warmth the butter.

3.   Pour ¼ of the egg mixture into your skillet.

4.   After that, cook for two minutes per side.

5.   Repeat to use the whole batter.

6.   Serve warm and enjoy!

Nutrition (Per Serving)

Calories: 141

Fat: 11.5g

Carbohydrates: 0.6g

Protein: 8.9g

Cinnamon Baked Apple Chips

Serving: 2

Prep Time: 5 minutes

Cook Time: 2 hours

Ingredients:

1 teaspoon cinnamon

1-2 apples

How To:

1.   Preheat your oven to 200 degrees F.

2.   Take a pointy knife and slice apples into thin slices.

3.   Discard seeds.

4.   Line a baking sheet with parchment paper and arrange apples thereon.

5.   Confirm they are doing not overlap.

6.   Once done, sprinkle cinnamon over apples.

7.   Bake within the oven for 1 hour.

8.   Flip and bake for an hour more until not moist.

9.   Serve and enjoy!

Nutrition (Per Serving)

Calories: 147

Fat: 0g

Carbohydrates: 39g

Protein: 1g

Herb and Avocado Omelet

Serving: 2

Prep Time: 2 minutes

Cook Time: 10 minutes

Ingredients:

3 large free-range eggs

½ medium avocado, sliced

½ cup almonds, sliced

Salt and pepper as needed

How To:

1.   Take a non-stick skillet and place it over medium-high heat.

2.   Take a bowl and add eggs, beat the eggs.

3.   Pour into the skillet and cook for 1 minute.

4.   Reduce heat to low and cook for 4 minutes.

5.   Top the omelet with almonds and avocado.

6.   Sprinkle salt and pepper and serve.

7.   Enjoy!

Nutrition (Per Serving)

Calories: 193

Fat: 15g

Carbohydrates: 5g

Protein: 10g

Classic Apple and Cinnamon Oatmeal

Serving: 4

Prep Time: 15 minutes

Cook Time: 7-9 hours

Ingredients:

1 apple, cored, peeled and diced

1 cup steel-cut oats

2 ½ cups unsweetened vanilla almond milk

2 tablespoons honey

½ teaspoon vanilla extract

1 teaspoon ground cinnamon

How To:

1.   Grease the Slow Cooker well.

2.   Add the listed ingredients to your Slow Cooker and stir.

3.   Cover with lid and cook on LOW for 7-9 hours.

4.   Serve and enjoy!

Nutrition (Per Serving)

Calories: 126

Fat: 3g

Carbohydrates: 25g

Protein: 3g

Blackberry Chicken Wings

Serving: 4

Prep Time: 35 minutes

Cook Time: 50minutes

Ingredients:

3 pounds chicken wings, about 20 pieces ½ cup blackberry chipotle jam Sunflower seeds and pepper to taste ½ cup water

How To:

1.   Add water and jam to a bowl and blend well.

2.   Place chicken wings during a zip bag and add two-thirds of the marinade.

3.   Season with sunflower seeds and pepper.

4.   Let it marinate for half-hour.

5.   Pre-heat your oven to 400 degrees F.

6.   Prepare a baking sheet and wire rack, place chicken wings in wire rack and bake for quarter-hour.

7.   Brush remaining marinade and bake for half-hour more.

8.   Enjoy!

Nutrition (Per Serving)

Calories: 502

Fat: 39g

Carbohydrates: 01.8g

Protein: 34g

Generous Lemon Dredged Broccoli

Serving: 4

Prep Time: 10 minutes

Cook Time: 15 minutes

Ingredients:

2 heads broccoli, separated into florets

2 teaspoons extra virgin olive oil

1 teaspoon sunflower seeds

½ teaspoon pepper

1 garlic clove, minced

½ teaspoon lemon juice

How To:

1.   Pre-heat your oven to a temperature of 400 degrees F.

2.   Take an outsized sized bowl and add broccoli florets with some extra virgin vegetable oil, pepper, sea sunflower seeds and garlic.

3. Spread the broccoli call at one even layer on a fine baking sheet.

4. Bake in your pre-heated oven for about 15-20 minutes until the florets are soft enough to be pierced with a fork.

5. Squeeze juice over them generously before serving.

6. Enjoy!

Nutrition (Per Serving)

Calories: 49

Fat: 2g

Carbohydrates: 4g

Protein: 3g

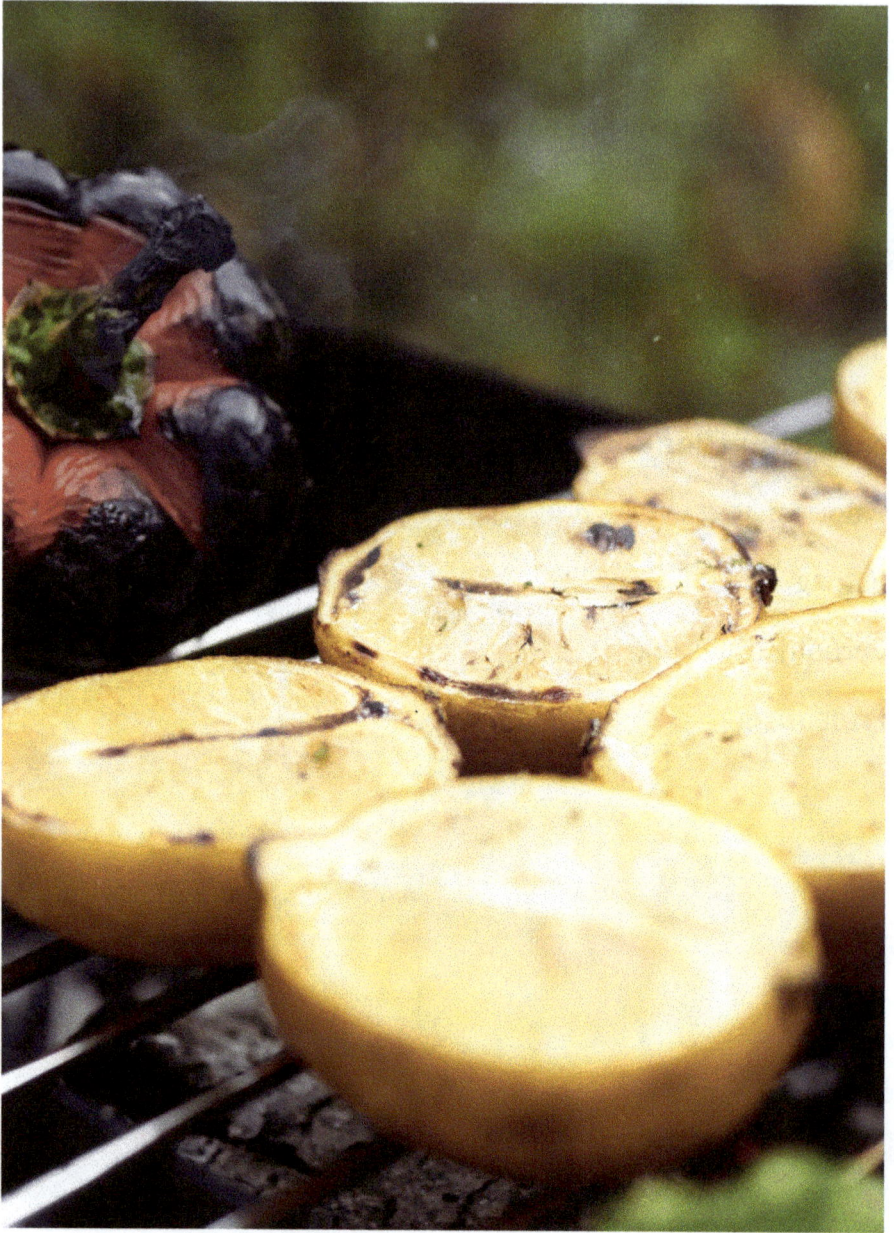

Tantalizing Almond butter Beans

Serving: 4

Prep Time: 5 minutes

Cook Time: 12 minutes

Ingredients:

2 garlic cloves, minced

Red pepper flakes to taste

Sunflower seeds to taste

2 tablespoons clarified butter

4 cups green beans, trimmed

How To:

1.   Bring a pot of water to boil, with added seeds for taste.

2.   Once the water starts to boil, add beans and cook for 3 minutes.

3.   Take a bowl of drinking water and drain beans, plunge them into the drinking water.

4.   Once cooled, keep them on the side.

5.   Take a medium skillet and place it over medium heat, add ghee and melt.

6.   Add red pepper, sunflower seeds, garlic.

7.   Cook for 1 minute.

8.   Add beans and toss until coated well, cook for 3 minutes.

9.   Serve and enjoy!

Nutrition (Per Serving)

Calories: 93

Fat: 8g

Carbohydrates: 4g

Protein: 2g

Healthy Chicken Cream Salad

Serving: 3

Prep Time: 5 minutes

Cook Time: 50 minutes

Ingredients:

2 chicken breasts

1 ½ cups low fat cream

3 ounces celery

2-ounce green pepper, chopped

½ ounce green onion, chopped

½ cup low fat mayo

3 hard-boiled eggs, chopped

How To:

1.   Pre-heat your oven to 350 degrees F.

2.   Take a baking sheet and place chicken, cover with cream.

3.   Bake for 30-40 minutes.

4.   Take a bowl and blend within the chopped celery, peppers, onions.

5.   Chop the baked chicken into bite-sized portions.

6.   Peel and chop the hard-boiled eggs.

7.   Take an outsized salad bowl and blend in eggs, veggies and chicken.

8.   Toss well and serve.

9.   Enjoy!

Nutrition (Per Serving)

Calories: 415

Fat: 24g

Carbohydrates: 4g

Protein: 40g

Generously Smothered Pork Chops

Serving: 4

Prep Time: 10 minutes

Cook Time: 30 minutes

Ingredients:

4 pork chops, bone-in

2 tablespoons of olive oil

¼ cup vegetable broth

½ pound Yukon gold potatoes, peeled and chopped 1 large onion, sliced

2 garlic cloves, minced

2 teaspoon rubbed sage

1 teaspoon thyme, ground

Pepper as needed

How To:

1.   Pre-heat your oven to 350 degrees F.

2.   Take an outsized sized skillet and place it over medium heat.

3.   Add a tablespoon of oil and permit the oil to heat up.

4.   Add pork chops and cook them for 4-5 minutes per side until browned.

5.   Transfer chops to a baking dish.

6.   Pour broth over the chops.

7.   Add remaining oil to the pan and sauté potatoes, onion, garlic for 3-4 minutes.

8.   Take an outsized bowl and add potatoes, garlic, onion, thyme, sage, pepper.

9.   Transfer this mixture to the baking dish (wish pork).

10.   Bake for 20-30 minutes.

11.   Serve and enjoy!

Nutrition (Per Serving)

Calorie: 261

Fat: 10g

Carbohydrates: 1.3g

Protein: 2g

Black Eyed Peas and Spinach Platter

Serving: 4

Prep Time: 10 minutes

Cook Time: 8 hours

Ingredients:

1 cup black eyed peas, soaked overnight and drained

2 cups low-sodium vegetable broth

1 can (15 ounces) tomatoes, diced with juice

8 ounces ham, chopped

1 onion, chopped

2 garlic cloves, minced

1 teaspoon dried oregano

1 teaspoon salt

½ teaspoon freshly ground black pepper ½ teaspoon ground mustard 1 bay leaf

How To:

1.   Add the listed ingredients to your Slow Cooker and stir.

2.   Place lid and cook on LOW for 8 hours.

3.   Discard the herb.

4.   Serve and enjoy!

Nutrition (Per Serving)

Calories: 209

Fat: 6g

Carbohydrates: 22g

Protein: 17g

Humble Mushroom Rice

Serving: 3

Prep Time: 10 minutes

Cook Time: 3 hours

Ingredients:

½ cup rice

2 green onions chopped

1 garlic clove, minced

¼ pound baby Portobello mushrooms, sliced 1 cup vegetable stock

How To:

1.   Add rice, onions, garlic, mushrooms, stock to your Slow Cooker.

2.   Stir well and place lid.

3.   Cook on LOW for 3 hours.

4.   Stir and divide amongst serving platters.

5. Enjoy!

Nutrition (Per Serving)

Calories: 200

Fat: 6g

Carbohydrates: 28g

Protein: 5g

Sweet and Sour Cabbage and Apples

Serving: 4

Prep Time: 15 minutes

Cook Time: 8 hours

Ingredients:

¼ cup honey

¼ cup apple cider vinegar

2 tablespoons Orange Chili-Garlic Sauce

1 teaspoon sea salt

3 sweet tart apples, peeled, cored and sliced

2 heads green cabbage, cored and shredded

1 sweet red onion, thinly sliced

How To:

1. Take a little bowl and whisk in honey, orange-chili aioli , vinegar.

2.   Stir well.

3.   Add honey mix, apples, onion and cabbage to your Slow Cooker and stir.

4.   Close lid and cook on LOW for 8 hours.

5.   Serve and enjoy!

Nutrition (Per Serving)

Calories: 164

Fat: 1g

Carbohydrates: 41g

Protein: 4g

Delicious Aloo Palak

Serving: 6

Prep Time: 10 minutes

Cook Time: 6-8 hours

Ingredients:

2 pounds red potatoes, chopped

1 small onion, diced

1 red bell pepper, seeded and diced

¼ cup fresh cilantro, chopped

1/3 cup low-sodium veggie broth

1 teaspoon salt

½ teaspoon Garam masala

½ teaspoon ground cumin

¼ teaspoon ground turmeric

¼ teaspoon ground coriander

¼ teaspoon freshly ground black pepper 2 pounds fresh spinach, chopped

How To:

1.   Add potatoes, bell pepper, onion, cilantro, broth and seasoning to your Slow Cooker.

2.   Mix well.

3.   Add spinach on top.

4.   Place lid and cook on LOW for 6-8 hours.

5.   Stir and serve.

6.   Enjoy!

Nutrition (Per Serving)

Calories: 205

Fat: 1g

Carbohydrates: 44g

Protein: 9g

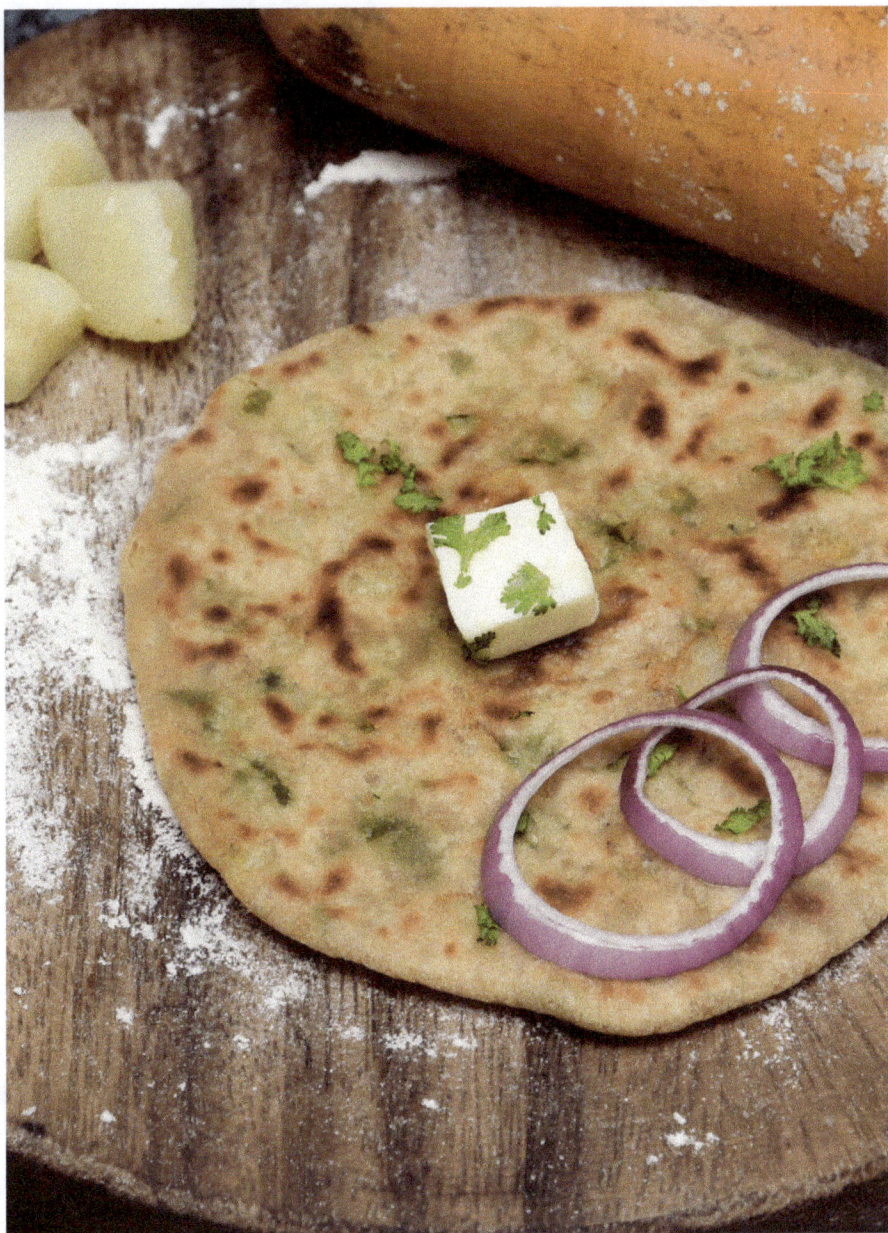

Healthy Mediterranean Lamb Chops

Serving: 4

Prep Time: 10 minutes

Cook Time: 10-minute

Ingredients:

4 lamb shoulder chops, 8 ounces each

2 tablespoons Dijon mustard

2 tablespoons Balsamic vinegar

½ cup olive oil

2 tablespoons shredded fresh basil

How To:

1.   Pat your lamb chops dry using a kitchen towel and arrange them on a shallow glass baking dish.

2.   Take a bowl and whisk in Dijon mustard, balsamic vinegar, pepper and mix them well.

3.   Whisk in the oil very slowly into the marinade until the mixture is smooth.

4.   Stir in basil.

5.   Pour the marinade over the lamb chops and stir to coat both sides well.

6.   Cover the chops and allow them to marinate for 1-4 hours (chilled).

7.   Take the chops out and let them rest for 30 minutes to allow the temperature to reach a normal level.

8.   Pre-heat your grill to medium heat and add oil to the grate.

9.   Grill the lamb chops for 5-10 minutes per side until both sides are browned.

10.   Once the center reads 145 degrees F, the chops are ready, serve and enjoy!

Nutrition (Per Serving)

Calories: 521

Fat: 45g

Carbohydrates: 3.5g

Protein: 22g

A Turtle Friend Salad

Serving: 6

Prep Time: 5 minutes

Cook Time: 5 minutes

Ingredients:

1 Romaine lettuce, chopped

3 Roma tomatoes, diced

1 English cucumber, diced

1 small red onion, diced

½ cup parsley, chopped

2 tablespoons virgin olive oil

½ large lemon, juice

1 teaspoon garlic powder

Sunflower seeds and pepper to taste

How To:

1.   Wash the vegetables thoroughly under cold water.

2.   Prepare them by chopping, dicing or mincing as needed.

3.   Take a large salad bowl and transfer the prepped veggies.

4.   Add vegetable oil, olive oil, lemon juice, and spice.

5.   Toss well to coat.

6.   Serve chilled if preferred.

7.   Enjoy!

Nutrition (Per Serving)

Calories: 200

Fat: 8g

Carbohydrates: 18g

Protein: 10g

Avocado and Cilantro Mix

Serving: 2

Prep Time: 10 minutes

Cook Time: nil

Ingredients:

2 avocados, peeled, pitted and diced

1 sweet onion, chopped

1 green bell pepper, chopped

1 large ripe tomato, chopped

¼ cup of fresh cilantro, chopped

½ lime, juiced

Sunflower seeds and pepper as needed

How To:

1.   Take a medium sized bowl and add onion, tomato, avocados, bell pepper, lime and cilantro.

2.   Give the whole mixture a toss.

3.   Season accordingly and serve chilled.

4.   Enjoy!

Nutrition (Per Serving)

Calories: 126

Fat: 10g

Carbohydrates: 10g

Protein: 2g

Exceptional Watercress and Melon Salad

Serving: 4

Prep Time: 15 minutes

Cook Time: 20 minutes

Ingredients:

3 tablespoons lime juice

1 teaspoon date paste

1 teaspoon fresh ginger root, minced

¼ cup vegetable oil

2 bunch watercress, chopped

2 ½ cups watermelon, cubed

2 ½ cups cantaloupe, cubed

1/3 cup almonds, toasted and sliced

How To:

1.   Take a large sized bowl and add lime juice, ginger, date paste.

2.   Whisk well and add oil.

3.   Season with pepper and sunflower seeds.

4.   Add watercress, watermelon.

5.   Toss well

6.   Transfer to a serving bowl and garnish with sliced almonds.

7.   Enjoy!

Nutrition (Per Serving)

Calories: 274

Fat: 20g

Carbohydrates: 21g

Protein: 7g

Zucchini and Onions Platter

Serving: 4

Prep Time: 15 minutes

Cook Time: 45 minutes

Ingredients:

3 large zucchini, julienned

1 cup cherry tomatoes, halved

½ cup basil

2 red onions, thinly sliced

¼ teaspoon sunflower seeds

1 teaspoon cayenne pepper

2 tablespoons lemon juice

How To:

1.   Create zucchini Zoodles by using a vegetable peeler and shaving the zucchini with peeler lengthwise until you get to the core and seeds.

2.   Turn zucchini and repeat until you have long strips.

3. Discard seeds.

4. Lay strips in cutting board and slice lengthwise to your desired thickness.

5. Mix Zoodles in a bowl alongside onion, basil, tomatoes and toss.

6. Sprinkle sunflower seeds and cayenne pepper on top.

7. Drizzle lemon juice.

8. Serve and enjoy!

Nutrition (Per Serving)

Calories: 156

Fat: 8g

Carbohydrates: 6g

Protein: 7g

Tender Watermelon and Radish Salad

Serving: 4

Prep Time: 15 minutes

Cook Time: 25 minutes

Ingredients:

medium beets, peeled and cut into 1-inch chunks 1 teaspoon extra virgin olive oil 4 cups seedless watermelon, diced

1 tablespoon fresh thyme, chopped

1 lemon, juiced

2 cups kale, torn

3 cups radish, diced

Sunflower seeds, to taste

Pepper, to taste

How To:

1.   Pre-heat your oven to 350 degrees F.

2.   Take a small bowl and add beets, olive oil and toss well to coat the beets.

3.   Roast beets for 25 minutes until tender.

4.   Transfer to large bowl and cool them.

5.   Add watermelon, kale, radishes, thyme, lemon juice, and toss.

6.   Season sea sunflower seeds and pepper.

7.   Serve and enjoy!

Nutrition (Per Serving)

Calories: 178

Fat: 2g

Carbohydrates: 39g

Protein: 6g

Fiery Tomato Salad

Serving: 4

Prep Time: 10 minutes

Cook Time: 25 minutes

Ingredients:

½ cup scallions, chopped

1 pound cherry tomatoes

3 teaspoons olive oil

Sea sunflower seeds and freshly ground black pepper, to taste 1 tablespoon red wine vinegar

How To:

1.   Season tomatoes with spices and oil.

2.   Heat your oven to 450 degrees F.

3.   Take a baking sheet and spread the tomatoes.

4.   Bake for 15 minutes.

5.   Stir and turn the tomatoes.

6.   Then, bake again for 10 minutes.

7.   Take a bowl and mix the roasted tomatoes with all the remaining ingredients.

8.   Serve and enjoy!

Nutrition (Per Serving)

Calories: 115

Fat: 10.4g

Carbohydrates: 5.4g

Protein: 12g

Spiced Up Salmon

Serving: 4

Prep Time: 10 minutes

Cook Time: 10 minutes

Ingredients:

Salmon fillets

2 tablespoons olive oil

1 teaspoon cumin, ground

1 teaspoon sweet paprika

1 teaspoon chili powder

½ teaspoon garlic powder

Pinch of pepper

How To:

1.   Take a bowl and add cumin, paprika, onion, chili powder, garlic powder, pepper and toss well.

2.   Rub the salmon in the mixture.

3.   Take a pan and place it over medium heat, add oil and let it heat up.

4.   Add salmon and cook for 5 minutes, both sides.

5.   Divide between plates and serve.

6.   Enjoy!

Nutrition (Per Serving)

Calories: 220

Fat: 10g

Net Carbohydrates: 8g

Protein: 10g

Coconut Cream Shrimp

Serving: 4

Prep Time: 10 minutes

Cook Time: nil

Ingredients:

1 pound shrimp, cooked, peeled and deveined

1 tablespoon coconut cream

¼ teaspoon jalapeno, chopped ½ teaspoon lime juice 1 tablespoon parsley, chopped Pinch of pepper

How To:

1.   Take a bowl and add shrimp, cream, jalapeno, lime juice, parsley, pepper.

2.   Toss well and divide into small bowls.

3.   Serve and enjoy!

Nutrition (Per Serving)

Calories: 183

Fat: 5g

Net Carbohydrates: 12g

Protein: 8g

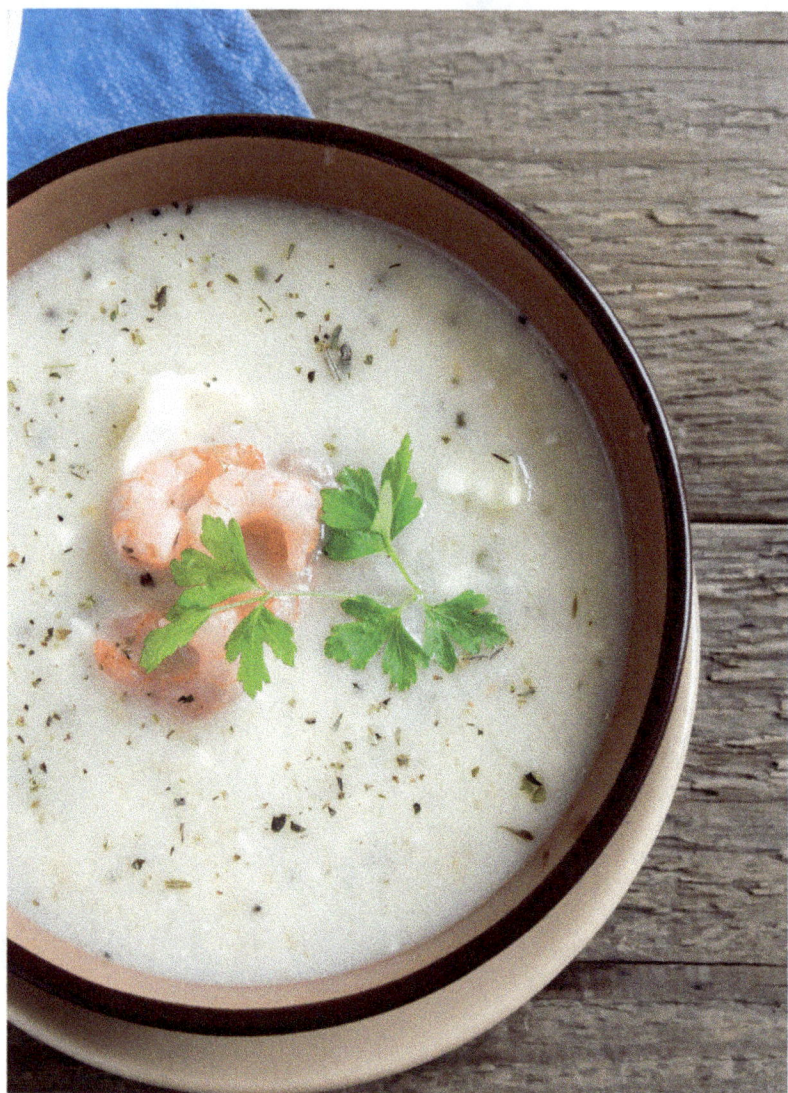

www.ingramcontent.com/pod-product-compliance
Lightning Source LLC
Chambersburg PA
CBHW050751030426
42336CB00012B/1756